SIMPLE KETO DIET FOR BEGINNERS

Lose Weight Fast: Lose 5 Pounds In 7 Days With This 7 Days Keto Diet Plan and Keto Top Tips For Beginners

DR. MICHAEL SAM

TABLE OF CONTENT

INTRODUCTION

Weight reduction can be a long journey for certain individuals yet in the event that you are searching for how to lose weight in a short space of time, this straightforward seven days keto diet plan for beginners will assist you with dropping weight rapidly.

It can trim the fats down fast in only seven days by following this seven-day meal plan and tips for quick weight loss.

CHAPTER ONE

Keto Diet 101: The Best Keto Diet

For Beginners

When starting an eating routine, it is normally best to make things basic for yourself. On the off chance that you are searching for a plan that assists with losing weight, burning fat and in any event, improving your health, the Keto diet is the ideal eating plan particularly when you have to drop weight rapidly.

If the basis of a keto diet which is high in fats and low in carbs sounds recognizable, you are correct.

Keto diet refers to a high fat and low carb diet that offers numerous medical benefits. The ketogenic diet is an eating plan that drives the body into ketosis, a state where the body utilizes fat as the essential fuel source (rather than starches).

In this special plan, you should eat under 25 grams net carbs a day for the body to accomplish fat-burning ketosis state.

The body turns out to be extraordinary at burning fat, and when the more reserved fat is utilized as a fuel, the more weight will be lost. It might sound bizarre to eat a high-fat diet regimen to burn excess fat and lose weight rapidly, yet the eating plan has been very much considered and proven. To put it plainly, any food that is high in carbs ought to be maintained a strategic distance from.

The objective of keto diet is to assist you with shedding pounds proficiently by getting to a metabolic state where your body burns fat rather than carbs and sugar. Keto diets have increased fat content, it is prohibitive, and are generally administered by an expert. However, this significant level of fat may not be compulsory for you to have the fat-burning condition of ketosis consistently.

Following an all-around defined keto diet plan with enough fiber from vegetables, moderate protein, just about 25 grams of net carbs or less every day, and up to 65% of your day by day calories are originating from healthy fats. The Keto diet guarantees proficient weight reduction results in about a short space of time.

CHAPTER TWO

Keto Diet Top Tips For Beginners

On the off chance that you are a newbie to the keto diet world, here are some simple tips to start your keto diet journey.

- **Decrease carbs (still eat a considerable measure of veggies)**

Eating a decreased amount of carb in the keto eating plan is important to accomplishing ketosis, however low carb doesn't mean no carb. After this beginning stage, you will gradually include little measures of net carbs once again into your eating regimen as you are burning fat.

When decreasing your carb intake on a keto diet plan to 20-30 net grams daily, it is important to eat a lot of vegetables to ensure you are getting the entirety of your essential nutrients and minerals, including fiber.

Go for nutrient dense veggies and veggies that are not starchy, for example, kale, spinach, asparagus, mushrooms and broccoli.

Top tip

The blend of eating an entire food and steadily including carbs as ketosis happens consistently, additionally assists with forestalling hunger sentiments and desires for processed food (food cravings).

Switch low carb ingredients to make your preferred meals. For example, you can utilize zucchini noodles to supplant customary noodles in your best pasta dish.

- **Diminish Stress**

We know that the vast majority of the occasions a reduced stress level, is more difficult to accomplish than one might expect! Increased degrees of the stress hormone cortisol can catapult your glucose levels and hold up traffic for your body's capacity to arrive at ketosis.

If your standard occupation or personal life is upsetting on an ordinary or on a normal, you are stressed every now and then, you might need to hold up a little to begin a keto diet.

You can likewise help in diminishing stressed by having lots of rest or sleep, practicing relaxation procedures, for example, yoga and the likes.

Top tip

Plan your sleep by following a set sleep time plan, and have an objective of 7-9 hours of sleep each night.

- **Increase Healthy Fats**

Low carb keto diet supplant your diminished amount of carbs with an increase fat content, which unquestionably represents at any rate 60% of your day by day calories intake. Since we were advised for a really long time to avoid fat, a great number of people under eat fat as they attempt keto diet.

It is basic to pick healthy fats from quality plant and creature sources like olive oil, coconut oil and avocado oil just as cheddar, eggs, fish and nuts.

Top tip

In the event that you see yourself getting ravenous after meals, the reason could be that you may not be eating adequate healthy fats.

- **Increase Work Out**

Similarly as with an eating regimen, increasing your working out levels or exercising daily can help you in accomplishing your weight loss objectives. Working out daily while on the keto diet can likewise assist you with accomplishing ketosis and transformation into a low carb, high fat way of life quickly than you can imagine. Reason being that, to accomplish ketosis, your body needs to eliminate any glucose, and as you exercise daily, the quicker your body exhausts its glycogen stores before converting it to fat for energy.

Top tip

It is not abnormal to feel somewhat slow as you start a keto diet. Ace any new exercise plan, and make certain to incorporate a lot of low power practices as you become accustomed to your new eating regimen.

- **Increase your Water Intake**

Water is essential to supporting your digestion and common body processes, and keto diets typically have a diuretic impact on the body. Not drinking enough water, particularly during the starting stage, can result to cravings, drowsiness and constipation.

As you drink enough water, ensure your body gets the entirety of your electrolytes by adding some stock to your eating regimen or extra salt to your meal.

Top tip

Stay all around hydrated and drink in any event 6 to 8 glasses of water each day. Drink more in the event that you have increased the degree of your activity or if the climate is hot.

• Keep up your protein consumption

A keto diet requires eating adequate protein to give the liver amino acids to make new glucose for the cells and organs, similar to your kidneys and your red blood cells, that can't utilize ketones or fatty acids as fuel.

Not having the option to eat adequate protein can result to loss of muscle, while consuming an extreme sum can forestall ketosis.

Top tip

When following a keto diet, target this percentage, 20-30% of your eating plan should consist of protein.

- **Keep up your Social activity**

Starting a keto diet doesn't mean you have to eat each food at home. Make legit decisions when eating out by checking the menu before you go there, request for the eatery nutrition data and go for meat and veggie choices, and a side serving of mixed greens is superior to a bland

fries.

Top tip

Swap sugar-loaded ingredients, for example,

BBQ sauce and ketchup with yellow mustard, hot

sauce ranch dressing, or margarine.

CHAPTER THREE

Foods To Avoid And Foods To Eat

Foods to Avoid

Sweet foods: Avoid fruit juice, cakes, frozen yogurt, desserts, smoothies, soda.

Grains or starches: rice, pasta, wheat based items, oat.

Fruits: Avoid all fruits aside from little portions of berries, for example, strawberries.

Beans or vegetables: kidney beans, peas, lentils, chickpeas.

Root vegetables and tubers: yams, parsnips, carrots, potatoes.

Low-fat products: These are enormously processed and generally high in carbs.

A few condiments or sauces: This normally contain sugar and undesirable fat.

Unhealthy fat: decrease your intake of processed vegetable oils and mayonnaise.

Liquor: Because of its carb content, numerous alcoholic drinks can move you out of ketosis.

Sugar free diet products: These are generally high in sugar alcohols, which can cause issues to ketone levels at times. These foods have been seen as enormously processed moreover.

Foods to Eat

Meat: Eat ham, wiener, steak, bacon, chicken, red meat and turkey.

Fatty fish: like fish, salmon, mackerel and trout.

Eggs: Search for fed or omega-3 entire eggs.

Spread and cream: search for grass-fed whenever the situation allows.

Cheddar: Unprocessed cheese (goat, cream, cheddar blue or mozzarella).

Nuts and seeds: such as walnuts, almonds, pumpkin seeds, flaxseeds, chia seeds.

Healthy oils: For example, extra virgin olive oil, avocado oil and coconut oil

Avocados: You can go for newly made guacamole or full avocados

Low-carb veggies: For example, most green veggies, onions, tomatoes peppers.

Condiments: You can utilize salt, pepper and a few solid herbs and flavors.

When you need to lose weight, you should

base the vast majority of your meals around these

foods.

CHAPTER FOUR

The Best Simple 7 Days Keto Diet Plan

There are numerous examinations that shows that a Keto diet can assist one with getting more fit, improve their wellbeing and wellness. Notwithstanding, accomplishing the state of Ketosis, you have to follow a simple keto diet plan. This plan will assist you with losing weight efficiently and rapidly, with this plan, it is certain you are losing 5 pounds in 7 days. Truly, it is very much possible.

Day 1:

Breakfast: Take easy egg salad

Snack: Take a bunch of cashew nuts

Lunch: Take spicy chicken sauté with avocado

Snack: Eat hard boiled egg

Dinner: Mini courgette with avocado burgers

Day 2:

Breakfast: Keto ground pork and fried eggs (scrambled)

Snack: Take a moderate quantity of almonds

Lunch: Eat pepper cabbage hamburger rolls

Snack: Go for 2 cuts of turkey

Dinner: Take pork chops and green apple radish salsa with broccoli slaw

Day 3:

Breakfast: Eat baked spicy avocado and eggs

Snacks: Take turkey jerky (look for no additional sugar type)

Lunch: Take lemon dark pepper tuna salad

Snack: Take 1 oz. cheddar and celery

Dinner: Eat spinach bacon sauté with avocado mint soup

Day 4:

35 | Page

Breakfast: Take an energy boosting keto rich smoothie

Snack: Go for 2 Tbsp. sun butter

Lunch: Eat turkey and dandelion greens with chicory salad

Snack: Eat cocoa almond fat bombs

Dinner: Take roasted rosemary beef tenderloin

Day 5:

Breakfast: Go for keto egg cake

Snack: Use 2 Tbsp. almond spread with celery sticks

Lunch: Eat keto lemon dark pepper fish salad

Snack: Take moderate quantity of cashew nuts

Dinner: Eat pork chops with green apple radish salsa and broccoli slaw

Day 6:

Breakfast: Eat plain porridge meal

Snack: Take a bunch of cashew nuts

Lunch: Go for Keto tamari marinated steak salad

Snack: Use 2 Tbsp of sun margarine and celery

Dinner: Take keto simple fajitas with simpler guacamole

Day 7:

Breakfast: Eat avocado with eggs Porridge

Snack: Use 1 oz. cheddar and a bunch of blueberries

Lunch: Go for keto coconut chicken strips

Snack: Eat hard boiled egg

Dinner: Take ground meat and courgette stew